BRAIN AND LANGUAGE

NEW YORK UNIVERSITY
SLAVIC PAPERS
(Interdisciplinary Studies)

EDITOR:
ANDREJ KODJAK
New York University

Volume IV

ROMAN JAKOBSON
with the assistance of
Kathy Santilli

BRAIN AND LANGUAGE

Cerebral Hemispheres and Linguistic Structure in Mutual Light

1980

Slavica Publishers, Inc.

Columbus, Ohio

For a complete catalog of Slavica books, with prices and ordering information, write to:
Slavica Publishers, Inc.
P.O. Box 14388
Columbus, Ohio 43214.

ISBN: 0-89357-068-0.

Typography by Brevis Press, Cheshire, Connecticut.

Printed in the United States of America by Thomson-Shore, Inc., Dexter, Michigan 48130.

EDITOR'S NOTE

Roman Jakobson's lecture "Brain and Language" given at New York University, May 6, 1980, is, as its title indicates, of primary interest to students of the medical sciences, linguistics, and neurolinguistics, but it also penetrates the areas of fundamental problems in poetics, general literary studies, and semiotics. Because of the last aspect of this work, the author gave us his most generous consent to include the present study in our series *New York University Slavic Papers, Interdisciplinary Studies*. For this we are profoundly grateful.

For the swift publication of the present volume we want to express our appreciation to Professor Charles Gribble, President of Slavica Publishers, and to Ms. Brenda Jubin of Brevis Press.

BRAIN AND LANGUAGE

I

Disruptions of language, and especially of its sound pattern, all those provoked by diverse brain lesions, have posed a number of interdisciplinary questions point-blank and brought aphasia into the basic program of my studies in a manner parallel with the opposite and nevertheless cognate phenomena of language acquisition. Those structural laws which govern the aphasic impairments of language were a problem cursorily pointed out in my address for the Fifth International Congress of Linguists which was to have been held in Brussels, September 1939 (see Jakobson 1962, 317ff.).

In a paper presented at the Ciba Foundation Symposium on disorders of language (London, May 1963), I attempted to outline the linguistic viewpoint on aphasia and to defend the need for a classification of aphasic syndromes to be based on "thoroughly integrated medical and linguistic research." The study of aphasia could no longer bypass the pertinent fact that an intrinsically linguistic typology of aphasic detriments, drafted without regard to the anatomical data, yielded nonetheless a surprisingly coherent relational pattern remarkably close to the topography of those cerebral lesions which underlie these impairments. The three linguistic dichotomies of aphasic losses unwittingly approached the sixfold table of cerebral damages delineated by the prominent psychoneurologist A. R. Luria (cf. Jakobson 1962, 289ff.). For the science of language these gradually emerging correspondences between the neural and linguistic fundamentals of an aphasic typology put an end to the randomly monistic "antilocalizationist theories" which strove to reduce the various types of aphasia to mere degrees of one single ailment (cf. Maruszewski, 35ff.; Luria 1974). The question of the interconnection between the topography of the brain and the structure of language supplied the joint, coordinated research of the early sixties with new and wider outlooks.

II

As was singled out in the concluding remarks at the Symposium on the Models for the Perception of Speech and Visual Form held in Boston, October 1964 (see Jakobson 1971, 338), Donald Broadbent (1954) suggested and Doreen Kimura (1961) widely developed unusual experiments in dichotic hearing: a simultaneous two-channel reception of diverse auditory stimuli by the two ears. These tests proved that the right ear displays a better aptitude for a precise recognition of speech sounds, while the left differs from the right in exhibiting an efficient discrimination of all other acoustic units. (For references see Peuser, 250: Dichotomous Stimulation). The privileged status of speech sounds in the right ear reveals the lateral pathway leading to the left hemisphere, as it was vividly brought up in the discussion. We are facing the substantial problem of assessing and explaining the difference between the speech components dependent on the left hemisphere and all other audible stimuli tied exclusively to the right side of the brain. The discrimination between those central mechanisms controlling the linguistic sphere proper and those processing the perception and comprehension of all other sounds, whether produced by the human organs or of some extrinsic origin, was for a long time underestimated, disregarded, or even denied, whereas today the phonetic trend, preoccupied solely with the speech sounds, becomes distinctly delimited from the nonspeech motor and acoustic domain.

At present the gradually observed essential difference between the particular cerebral treatment of speech on the one hand and the rest of the auditory phenomena on the other hand calls for a further, much more comprehensive and specific scrutiny.

In addition to numerous medical examinations of patients "with stable, unilateral cortical lesions" (cf. Brenda Milner 1975, 7), the ensuing progress in the investigation of the separate hemispheres profited from the split-brain experience connected with the section of the cerebral commissures, an operation practiced on epileptics since the 1960's (cf. Gazzaniga & Sperry 1967; Gazzaniga 1970; Sperry 1975). The conclusions drawn from these operations confirmed the intimate ties linking speech (and also at least certain varieties of writing and calculation) precisely with the left hemisphere—and what was particularly instructive—the connection between higher verbal processes and the left, dominant hemisphere. This connection proved instrumental in opening new insights into the structuration of language.

And now, unilateral electroconvulsive therapy (ECT),

practiced on schizophrenic and on depressive patients, has been used in a most imaginative way to provide for the first time systematic data about brain and language in humans without fixed brain lesions. As the only preliminary effort in the same direction we may quote the Sodium Anytal injections reported by Milner (1975, 84f.) and used to inactivate both hemispheres in turn. The fact that a unilateral ECT produces a short-term disruption of one hemisphere, a deficit followed by a gradual return to the normal state, permits comparisons never before feasible on such a scale. The procedure, developed since the late 1960's in some Russian medical centers, has been recently accompanied by minute and keen observations on changes in status and behavior after the unilateral shock.

Since the early 1960's the technique of unilateral electroconvulsive therapy underwent a considerable development (see, e.g. Cannicott 1963; Halliday et al.), but the functional difference between the left- and right-sided shock lacked until recently any intense and systematic consideration. Meanwhile, the temporal inactivation of one of the two hemispheres, depending upon the direction of the electric shock, results in opposite effects on the auditory as well as on the motor experiences of the patient.

For the preliminary evidence of this persistently progressing inquiry, see first and foremost the valuable publications sponsored by the Sečenov Institute of Evolutionary Physiology and Biochemistry at the

Academy of Sciences (*Akademija Nauk* = AN) of the U.S.S.R.: the first, *Hearing and Speech of the Dominant and Nondominant Hemispheres,* written jointly by Balonov and Deglin (1976), and the second, *Unilateral Electroconvulsive Shock,* by the same authors and a few collaborators (1979). Substantial contributions to this research have been made by the eminent Russian expert in the science of language, Vjačeslav Ivanov, especially in his book *Even and Odd: the Asymmetry of the Brain and of Sign Systems* (1978) and in a later Tartu essay, "Semiotics of Oral Speech and the Functional Asymmetry of the Brain" (1979). Cf. also Bragina's and Dobroxotova's Russian book, *Functional Asymmetry and Psychopathology of the Focal Affections of the Brain* (1977) with its instructive perusal of the comparative inquiry into the relationship of the cerebral hemispheres.

Norman Geschwind's (1979) vigilant inquiry into the dependence of higher activities such as language "on specialized regions of the human brain" opens new vital questions for interdisciplinary research. While a linguist is obliged to stop at the functional asymmetry of the brain, Geschwind's rich neurological experience enables him to touch also upon the arresting questions of the material, anatomic divergence between the two hemispheres (cf. Geschwind, 196; Galaburda et al. 1978).

III

After having outlined jointly with Linda Waugh a set of preliminary remarks and issues in *The Sound Shape of Language* (1979), the next step I would venture is a tentative answer to the question of the general criteria which separate the two spheres of auditory stimuli from each other—those processed by the left and those by the right hemisphere of the brain. The bifurcated cerebral localization of the two realms of constituents is so manifest that the question of those properties which encompass and unify each of the two varieties and discriminate them from each other inevitably arises.

First the varied experiments with dichotic hearing, second the evidence received from patients with split-brain operations, third the examination of patients with one hemisphere damaged, and fourth and foremost the comparative study of the temporary role played by the electroshocks when inactivating one of the hemispheres, all these sources agree in defining the exact range of the phenomena controlled by the left and those by the right hemisphere.

The disturbances of the sound pattern prove to be

most rigorous in the abolishment of one-feature distinctions between phonemes (cf. Balonov, Baru, & Deglin 1975). The impoverishment and demolition of the phonemic, especially consonantal repertory sets in briefly after the shock, and the gradual reappearance of the former, habitual constitution takes from ten or twenty minutes to an hour and a half (see *AN* 1979, 70f. and 87). The relative chronology of this restitution should be thoroughly traced, as it had been suggested forty years ago at the Uppsala observations of the patients' verbal recovery from insulin shocks (see now Jakobson & Waugh, 34). In this way new data could be attained for the ever timely question of similarities between the gradual restitution of ECT patients' speech and the progressive acquisition of children's language.

IV

The primary informative task of the ultimate components of language, the distinctive features and their bundles into phonemes, requires a mediate, even a multi-mediate relation among them before these elementary quanta, entities lacking by themselves "any singleness of reference" (see Sapir, *Selected Writings*, 34) and designating nothing but mere otherness, appear organized into a cohesive referential complex. This network of language is under the full control of the left hemisphere. As Balonov & Deglin conclude in the tenth, final chapter of their basic volume (*AN* 1976, 182), "it appears evident that as a rule the left hemisphere carries out the classification of phonemes by proceeding from the distinctive features, supports the hierarchy of these features, and ensures herewith the stability of the language's phonological system." In its turn, the process of inactivation undergone by the left hemisphere reveals a set of correspondences with the rules which underlie the ensuing disintegration of the given phonological system, on its auditory as well as motor level: cf. *AN* 1976 (133, 136, 181f.) and *AN* 1979 (103). As examples of symmetry between the dissolution of the vocalic and consonantal patterns one may quote the relative stability of the poles of compactness — /a/ and /k/ and the parallel merger of tonality pairs such as /u/ — /i/ and /p/ — /t/.

The even more mediate character of contextual, redundant features furthers the increase of their dependence on the left cerebral hemisphere. The frequently increasing scarcity of redundant variations in the speech of subjects with a temporal inactivation of the left hemisphere is a linguistic event demanding a heightened attention of inquirers.

V

In contradistinction to the many-tiered involvement of the linguistic elements totally dependent on the intact activity of the left hemisphere, those sound phenomena which demand an unimpaired functioning of the right hemisphere all have in common one noticeable trait: they display a direct, immediate, ostensive relation between their external, material form and what is signaled. Our perception of speech sounds demands an apprehension of the sound pattern and of its cognitive functioning in a given language, whereas the identification of any nonspeech sound requires an immediate recognition of the stimulus perceived, its identification in form and meaning.

Both the experiments with dichotic hearing and the testimonies received from patients subjected to unilateral electroshocks have shown again and again the indispensable connection linking all these varied percepts with the underlying activity of the right hemisphere. "Environmental noises such as a car starting, the sharpening of a pencil, water running, and oral emissions apart from speech—coughing, crying, laughing, humming, yawning, snoring, sniffling, sighing, panting or sobbing" were quoted as percepts controlled by the right hemisphere. Briefly, the latter processes any immediate audible manifestation of human and animal physiology and daily life, as well as motions stirred by the forces of nature (cf. Knox & Kimura 1970; King & Kimura 1972; Balonov & Deglin 1977).

The allegiance of one, superficially similar sound to two different cerebral hemispheres is, one could say, prompted by Sapir's introductory discussion to his epochal "Sound Patterns of English" (see 33ff.) where he compares two physically more or less similar formations—the candle-blowing sound and the prevocalic *wh* of such words as *when*—the former "'a *directly* functional act', while the latter has *no direct* functional value, it is merely a link in the construction of a symbol": "in brief, the candle-blowing *wh* means business; the speech sound *wh* is stored-up play which can eventually fall in line in a game that merely refers to business." The former is obviously processed by the right, and the latter by the left hemisphere.

To return once more to the Russian observations made in unilateral shock therapy, "subjects with a temporarily inactivated right hemisphere were helpless when faced with a succession of distinct auditory stimuli which were perfectly recognizable as long as this hemisphere maintained its activity: the tinkling of bells, singing birds, splashing water, neighing horses, a howling snowstorm, a roaring lion, a crying child, a clatter of crockery, peals of thunder, a grunting pig, the clank of metal, the call of a rooster, a barking dog, a lowing cow, the sound of a furnace, a passerby's footsteps, a cooing dove, the rumble of a plane, cackling geese, a ringing telephone, the roar of waves at high tide. During the inactivation of the right hemisphere, the noise of applause was actually taken for the winnowing of grain, laughter for crying, a thunderstorm for an engine, the squeal of a pig for the noise of a Caterpillar tractor, the honking of geese for the croaking of frogs, a dog barking for the cackling of hens, the noise of a motorcycle for that of an animal" (see *AN* 1976, Ch. 5; Jakobson & Waugh, 34f.).

VI

A peculiar place belongs to elements which permeate speech yet share the character of what one may call immediate signals. These particular ingredients of current discourse, listed loosely, without consistent delimitation, as interjections, exclamations, and ejaculations, stand outside the general syntactic patterning of language, and they are neither words nor sentences. They tend to differ from the phonological rules of usual vocabulary and semantically they are reduced to stereotyped affective expressions.

As John Hughlings Jackson comments in his renowned essay of 1874 on the nature of brain duality (135), "the communist orator did not really make a blunder when he began his oration '*Thank God* I'm an atheist,' for the expression *Thank God* is used by careless, vulgar people simply as an interjection, there being no thought at all about the primitive meaning." According to Jackson, "such ejaculations are verbal utterances more automatic than speech." It is characteristic that these zero parts of speech get easily misinterpreted or simply lost by subjects with a fully active left but simultaneously inactivated right hemisphere. The same situation frequently befalls violent swearing or cursing words and, on the other hand, endearments and other ritualized formulas of a courtly etiquette. A similar plight embraces numerous parasitic elements such as "hem," and the slight, deliberate sound of a cough amid an utterance (cf. Ivanov 1979, 131).

The second section of the "Introduction" to Trubetzkoy's *Grundzüge der Phonologie* is entitled "Phonologie und Lautstilistik" and attempts to delineate the difference between phonological, sense-discriminatory components proper and those stylistic modifications of speech sounds or of their sequences in discourse "by means of which emotionally tinged speech is distinguished from emotionally neutral, tranquil speech," either without any specification of the underlying emotion (e.g. German *schön* with a smaller or larger prolongation of the initial sibilant and with an additionally protracted vowel) or carrying a closer specification of the emotion meant, as for instance a tremor which is meant to render a feeling of fear. In both cases there is a thoroughly ostensive, immediate relation between the emotion and the means of signaling it. Such immediacy is a firm condition requiring the control of the right hemisphere, "mute" as well as "emoting" (Sperry, 11). A subject without an activation of the right hemisphere is liable to avoid any emotive ingredients, whereas the enactment of the right hemisphere makes the emotional shades of speech particularly apprehensible. Whatever common sound properties may be shared by the phonemic and emotive patterns of language, the dissimilar character of their use and their different cerebral location strikingly separate these two kinds of phenomena from each other.

When examining the role of the diverse emotives in speech, one must take into account Geschwind's judicious reminder (1979, 192) that the right hemisphere makes an important contribution to emotion and state of mind: "Lesions in the right hemisphere not only give rise to inappropriate emotional responses to the patient's own condition, but also impair his recognition of emotions in others. A patient with damage on the left side may not be able to comprehend a statement but in many cases he can still recognize the emotional tone with which it is pronounced. A patient with a disorder of the right hemisphere usually understands the meaning of what is said, but he often fails to recognize that it is spoken in an angry or a humorous way."

The inactivation of the right hemisphere imparts a monotonous, affectless character to the patient's utterances, and he loses the capacity of regulating his own voice in accordance with emotional situations. On the other hand, the reduction of the emotive ingredients leads the patient to a greater talkativeness. Thus the damping influence of the active right hemisphere moderates the verbal activity of the left hemisphere and increases the readability of the linguistic components. In these regards both hemispheres act in concert. One might recall that over one hundred years ago scientific intuition enabled the sagacious J. H. Jackson—especially in his essay of 1874—to assign the intellectual language to the left, and the emotional to the right hemisphere (see 1958, p. 134). Already in 1866 the earliest of Jackson's notes on the physiology and pathology of language opens with the statement that "there are two modes of expression, the emotional and the intellectual" (see 1958, 121).

VII

The recent observations of speech in connection with unilateral electric shocks brought to light new substantial proofs for the considerable independence of the sentential and, in particular, emotionally colored intonations. They emerge before children's acquisition of the sound pattern of their mother tongue, and in many aphasic instances we are faced with a mutual independence of such intonations and word phonology. The use of affirmative, interrogative, and avowedly emotional intonations outside of speech proper, or in mere mumbling sequences, provides additional proof for the autonomous occurrence of, so to say, extralinguistic intonational differences.

The experiments with dichotic hearing revealed the connection of such intonations solely with the right, yet by no means with the left hemisphere. Balonov's & Deglin's communications (*AN* 1976, 171ff.) comprehensively show the independence of such kinds of intonations from the left hemisphere and place their appearance, clear perceptibility, and reproducibility under the normal activity of the right hemisphere: "In the period of the right hemisphere's inactivation the identification of intonations sharply worsens." All the data obtained find their obvious explanation in the immediacy of the signal value displayed by these intonations which serve, so to speak, as period, comma, question mark, exclamation point, or ellipsis.

The inactivation of the right hemisphere leads to a deficit in ostensive communication. In semiotic literature (see especially Osolsobě) this way of communication might be defined as "placing something at the disposal of the cognitive activity of the person." A couple of shorts and socks exposed in a window announces a haberdasher's shop. Ostension merges with synecdoche: the voice of a patient's wife, which he hears without seeing her, is her *pars pro toto,* just as the sound and/or grimace of yawning is an ostensive, synecdochic expression of the simulated or natural drowsiness of a fatigued or bored utterer. The presence of an emotive tint in the speech sounds introduces an immediate information of the speaker's excitement into his message.

VIII

In contradistinction to the left hemisphere, the right one secures the ability of the patient to identify such auditory signals as the voices of his acquaintances when he hears their speech without seeing them, whereas the subject with an inactivated right and active left hemisphere is unable to recognize the most familiar voices, even those of his wife and children, and he does not grasp the transition from one speaker to another. Briefly, all audible physiognomic symptoms cease to work for him, even such general ones as the recognition of the difference between male and female voices. Also the question of the spatial source and direction of the voice heard is left unsolved: "Thus the spatial hearing remains unaltered after left-sided shocks but appears disturbed after right-sided ones" (*AN* 1979, 91).

The chief ability of the right hemisphere in the handling of auditory percepts is their immediate change into a simple, concrete concept lying outside of language proper, disclosing the nearest contiguous source of the sound stimulus produced and heard.

The comparative analysis of speech samples generated and/or perceived during the inactivation of one of the hemispheres has been hitherto concentrated primarily on the phonic level of language. The no less important morphological, syntactical, and lexical levels of such a comparison have not yet yielded sufficient material for exact conclusions and have not yet attracted the systematic attention of investigators.

With the inactivation of the left hemisphere the number of used and apprehended words and of their occurrences goes steadily down as does the variety and length of their syntactic combinations and subordination levels. "After left-sided unilateral shocks one observes a shift toward a range of elementary, superficial formations, whereas the right-sided shocks are followed by a shift toward complex multi-leveled constructions" (*AN* 1979, 75ff.).

The inactivation of the left hemisphere is particularly detrimental for verbs (except the simplest imperative formulas such as *stop* or *walk* or *help*) and for auxiliary words, while nominative forms of nouns, showing a much lower dependence on the context, are somewhat more under the control of the right hemisphere, especially when offering no complex word derivation, in particular no kinship with verbs. And finally, a higher resistability is exhibited by the most concrete and usual nouns (cf. Jakobson 1980, 104f.; on the intricate question of verb-derived nouns see Wolf & Koff 1970).

The immediacy of transition from the linguistic network to an extralinguistic reality makes a word less dependent upon the integrity of the left hemisphere. In this connection the extreme dependence of the so-called grammatical "shifters" (according to Jespersen's terminology) on the intact left hemisphere is most instructive, since the general meaning of a shifter comprises a simultaneous, double reference to the code and to the message (cf. Jakobson 1971, 130ff.). In contradistinction to the shifterless character of the noun, it is the compulsory participation of shifters in the structure of verbs which furthers an alienation between the verb and the right hemisphere. The vanishment of shifters from the range of grammatical categories and an atrophy of syntactic subordination are two characteristic effects called forth by the suppression of the left hemisphere.

Its inactivation underlies the desemantization of words on their paradigmatic as well as syntagmatic axis. Ivanov (1978, 39ff., 45) has initiated a promising study of the distinctions and confusions committed by patients under shock therapy between synonyms, antonyms, and homonyms. Changes in treatment of semantic similarities, contrasts, and contiguities in their relation to the withdrawal of single hemispheres promise to open new tempting outlooks.

The left hemisphere of the brain deals with categorization both in grammar and in the constructive operations of calculation (cf. Ivanov 1979, 126).

The captivating questions of the interconnection between script and cerebral hemispheres have been left aside in the present survey, in order not to embroil the discussion by including one more intricate, namely spatial factor.

The inquirers' find that "the entire scale of speech disturbances after the left-sided shocks appear much more frequently among depressive patients than among schizophrenics" (*AN* 1979, 69) asks for further observations and analysis.

IX

The scrutiny of the varied sound stimuli remains incomplete as long as one has not intently compared the case of speech sounds with another system of auditory signs, namely with musical elements. The frequent lack of concurrence between aphasia and amusia has been repeatedly observed and described. The aphasic loss of speech is often combined with a preserved or even developed ability to sing.

Milner's observations of patients with temporal lobectomies for epilepsy had evidenced the overwhelming concern of musical ability with the right hemisphere (1962), and Kimura's experiments in dichotic hearing came to support the same conclusion (1964). Kimura's "melodies test reconfirmed the finding, by then well established, of the left ear superiority/right hemisphere dominance" (Damásio, 146). The influence of unilateral shocks was keenly investigated by Balonov & Deglin (*AN* 1976, Ch. 5 and Table 21; cf. Mindadze et al.). The inactivation of the right hemisphere hinders both the identification of short musical phrases and the recognition of familiar melodies, as well as the reproduction of motifs heard, whereas the inactivation of the left hemisphere favors and furthers all such accomplishments. Briefly, the situation with musical sounds creates a syndrome basically similar to the treatment of nonspeech sounds and of the emotive ingredients in speech. The suppression of the right hemisphere may lead the patient as far as to a whimsical confusion between such dissimilar items as, for instance, the popular Russian song "Volga, Volga" and the melody of the rumba. The relative immediacy of musical perception explains the decisive role of the right hemisphere in the recognition, discrimination, and identification of phrases and melodies, as well as in their execution (Damásio, 151).

There is no doubt, however, that the question of musical perception still remains much less investigated than the various questions of verbal percepts and that several fundamental musical problems await further and deeper inquiry. The partial deviations from the dominance of the right hemisphere in regard to musical perception, which have been incidentally noticed (see Bever & Chiarello; Gates & Bradshaw), must advance the search for their delineation and final explanation. What must be particularly remembered is the variety of musical codes which imposes an obligation upon the explorer to learn to discount from his questionnaire all those elements which are out of the essentially musical perception of his examinees. In particular it is easy to comprehend why the similarity of accustomed, recalled melodies is more closely linked to the right hemisphere, in contradistinction to the recognizance of unfamiliar pieces, a procedure which unwittingly opens the question of their underlying code and therefore may attract the left hemisphere with its codifying specialization. The fundamental trait of musical signs, namely "*imputed* similarity," seems to be the true key to the unexpected, puzzling examples of their shift to the left hemisphere (cf. Jakobson 1980, 22ff.).

In the confrontation of music with language the comparison must be confined solely to language in its poetic function.

One should also mention the frequent confusion of examiners between disability to perceive music and to read notes; sometimes such a mix-up embroils the task of assigning music to one of the two hemispheres.

At last, we are met with a peculiar analogy: the right hemisphere manifests a greater ability and concentration in identifying musical phrases and/or melodies just in the case when the left hemisphere remains inactivated (*AN* 1979, 85ff.; Table 8.8), and this relation surprisingly corresponds to the greater talkativeness and verbal preciseness in speech of the left hemisphere when the right one is not working, as compared to the intact activity of both hemispheres.

X

In a stimulating paper devoted to "the functional asymmetry of the brain," Bragina & Dobroxotova have developed their view that the brain's hemispheres demonstrate different temporal orientations: "the right is turned into the past, the left into the future. . . . The left-side hemisphere is responsible for supplying abstract cognition. Sensitive cognition leans on the right space and on the past, whereas abstract cognition leans on the left space and on future time" (pp. 137, 146). The authors underscore that in contradistinction to the past, the future "has not yet been given for the subject's sensible experience and cannot serve as support for the formation of sensitive images."

These considerations find an unexpected, memorable, and well-grounded correspondence in the philosophical writings of Charles Sanders Peirce (cf. Jakobson 1980, 31ff.). In his contraposition of two kinds of signs, *icon* and *symbol,* the former is defined as "a representamen of what it represents and for the mind that interprets it as such, by virtue of its being as *immediate* image, that is to say by virtue of characters which belong to it in itself as a sensible object" (IV

#447). The mode of being of the symbol is, in Peirce's conception of this term, different from that of the icon. While the icon has such being as belongs to the *past* experience, the nature of a symbol, especially such as a verbal sign or the network of language, is the really working *general* rule. According to Peirce, "whatever is truly general refers to the indefinite future. . . . It is a potentiality; and its mode of being is *esse in futuro*" (II #148). "The value of a symbol is that it serves to make thought and conduct rational and enables us to predict the future" (IV #448).

Here lies the nucleus of an explanation for those "most surprising recent findings" which were pointed out by Geschwind (1979, 192): namely "behaviors denoting a catastrophic reaction or indicating an anxious-depressive orientation of mood" are particularly frequent among left brain-damaged patients, "chiefly in subjects with severe aphasia." Such reactions "appear generally after repeated failures in verbal communication" (Gainotti, 53).

Likewise the experience with unilateral electric shocks has confirmed the salient fact of "roughly expressed, negative emotions produced by the suppression of the left hemisphere" (Ivanov 1978, 107) and hence by the atrophy of verbal symbols. "The negative emotional shift" stirred up by the left-sided shock can drive the grief and sorrow of a depressive patient to "a nightmarish terror" (*AN* 1979, 96f.). The subject suffers from being deprived of the patterned symbols needed to program his future. It is with the functions of the "verbal hemisphere" that Ivanov connects "the realization of an individual as a single whole" (1979, 135).

The agnosia of symbolic rules and systems marks the inactivation of the left hemisphere. It occurs in an opposite sense if joined to the inactivation of the right hemisphere, and the consequent agnosia of ostension: when *res tota de parte* is no longer recognized by the subject.

The bipolar difference between these two opposite kinds of agnosia—in direct correspondence with the two contrary directions of the unilateral shocks—has found a telling illustration in the recent Russian report on the development of ECT (*AN* 1979, 92ff.). During the inactivation of the left hemisphere the patient loses his "formal" orientation in time based on the conventional codes of watch and calendar symbols but is prone to maintain the direct, subjective evaluation of the time run, whereas the right-side inactivation preserves the formal responses while abolishing the immediate subjective chronology.

The question of the interrelation between an active hemisphere and an inactivated one opens the way to comparisons between joint active hemispheres with individual variations as to their functional hierarchy; the significance of these individual variations for characterological studies is beyond any doubt.

XI

Two sets of questions are brought up by the progressing neurolinguistic research: first, the interhemispheric topics demand an ever closer linguistic, or to put it more exhaustively, semiotic approach; and secondly, we face a consistently interdisciplinary study of aphasic problems in connection with a difference in the affected zones of the left hemisphere. This inquiry, opened around the 1870's most tangibly by the medical experts — Paul Broca *1824–1880* (see 1888), J. H. Jackson *1835–1911* (see now 1958), and Carl Wernicke *1848–1905* (cf. Geschwind 1967, Eggert 1977) — still waits for new replies to the accumulated cruxes.

The experiments with unilateral electric shocks have already shown that this new technique can and will cast light not only on the interplay of both hemispheres, but also on the zonal subdivisions within the dominant (left) hemisphere, and on the correlative typology of aphasic impairments. As exemplified by Balonov & Deglin (*AN* 1976, 191), the left-side electric shocks, with respect to the placement of convulsive electrodes more backwards or forwards, patently help to elucidate the substantial difference between postero-temporal and fronto-temporal lesions of the brain, a distinction which finds its expression in two opposite linguistic syndromes of aphasia. In connection with the continuous development of varied clinical observations and trials, such a leading explorer in the analysis of traumatic aphasia as A. R. Luria in his studies of the seventies (see particularly 1973, 1974, and 1977) reached a final agreement with the earlier efforts on the linguistics side to delineate and explicate the dichotomous principles of aphasic disorders, even though "we don't yet know in detail the psychological features and physiological mechanisms underlying these impairments" (1973, 64).

Although at first glance these linguistic distinctions seemed to be "clinically insignificant" and although originally they found "no firm support in neurological characteristics," precisely the same linguistic distinctions have finally appeared to Luria as fundamental for the study of aphasia and at last "firmly supported by contemporary ideas of the functional organization of the human brain" (1977, 243). Thus the basic binary concepts viewed in the linguistic quest as the key to understanding the obvious dichotomy of aphasic disturbances, namely dyads such as Encoding/Decoding, Syntagmatic/Paradigmatic, and Continuity/Similarity (cf. Jakobson 1971, 229–259, 289–333; 1980, 93–111), gradually found access to the advanced neuropsychological treatment of aphasic enigmas.

At present those governing functions of the brain

which are connected with the output of speech and with its input lend themselves to an attentive examination, and it looks as if the joint efforts of linguists and neurologists are summoned to suggest and open ever deeper insights both into the structure of language with reference to the brain and into the structure of the brain with the help of language. The necessary initial step on this path has been the delineation of the set of internal functional convergences which specify each of the cerebral hemispheres; these two heterogenous sets prove to form a cardinal dichotomous system of diametrically opposite, while complementary properties, and such a state of affairs compels the maturing discipline of neurolinguistics to examine any display of one hemisphere with an unfailing reference to its counterpart on the other side of the brain.

It has been necessary to draw up a list of identifications and distinctions processed solely by the given hemisphere and inaccessible to the other hemisphere. The mutually exclusive stocks of the two hemispheres demand a clear delineation of the "many still rather ill-defined processes" which fall under the right hemisphere (cf. Milner 1975, 83), but actually the immediacy of their signification offers us the sought definition. Thus, e.g., the *mediacy* of phonological devices, such as a distinction of higher and lower pitch in a polytonic language like Thai, explains the dependence of this distinctive feature on the left hemisphere, as it has been proved by experiments with dichotic hearing and with unilateral shocks (cf. Jakobson & Waugh, 45). On the other hand, the *immediate* signification justifies the expected competence of the right hemisphere when for instance a higher pitch signals either an interrogative sentence or an emotive passage in the speaker's words, or finally the presence of a female's voice in the discourse.

To conclude with a telling case (cf. Monrad-Krohn 1947): A lesion of the left hemisphere, which was suffered by a Norwegian woman from a bomb fragment, cancelled the role of pitch in her native word pattern but released the latter's wider use in emotive variations to be processed by the right hemisphere. Each of the two signal systems—the immediate as well as the mediate one—is accessible to one single hemisphere: immediate signals can be processed only by the right hemisphere and the mediate by the left one.

To my friends Norman Geschwind and Allan Keiler, I'm indebted for their enlightening suggestions and considerations.

Cambridge, Mass.
April 1980

REFERENCES

AN (1976) = Akademija Nauk SSSR—Institut Èvoljucionnoj Fiziologii i Bioximii Imeni I. N. Sečenova, *Slux i reč' dominantnogo i nedominantnogo polušarij* by Balonov, Lev, & Vadim Deglin, Leningrad.

AN (1979) = Akademija Nauk etc., *Unilateral'nyj èlektrosudorožnyj pripadok* by Balonov, Lev, D. Barkan, & V. Deglin, Leningrad.

Balonov, L., A. Baru, & V. Deglin (1975), "Identifikacija sintezirovanyx glasnopodobnyx stimulov v uslovijax prexodjaščej inaktivacii dominantnogo i nedominantnogo polušarij," *Fiziologija čeloveka* 1, 395–404.

Balonov, L., & V. Deglin (1977), "Vosprijatie zvukovyx nerečevyx obrazov (sluxovoj i muzykal'nyj gnozis) v uslovijax inaktivacii dominantnogo i nedominantnogo polušarij," *Fiziologija čeloveka* 3, 415–423.

Bever, T. G., & R. Chiarello (1974), "Cerebral dominance in musicians and non-musicians," *Science* 185, 537–539.

Bragina, N. N., & T. A. Dobroxotova (1977), *Funkcional'naja asimmetrija i psixopatologija očagovyx poraženij mozga*, Moscow.

______ (1977), "Problema funkcional'noj asimmetrii mozga," *Voprosy filosofii* 2, 135–150.

Broadbent, D. E. (1954), "The Role of Auditory Localization in Attention and Memory," *Journal of Experimental Psychology* 47, 191–196.

Broca, P. (1888), *Mémoires sur le cerveau de l'homme,* Paris.

Cannicott, S. M. (1963), "The Technique of unilateral electroconvulsive therapy," *American Journal of Psychiatry* 120, 477–480.

Damásio, A. R., & Hanna Damásio (1977), "Musical Faculty and Cerebral Dominance," *Music and the Brain* ed. by M. Critchley et al., Springfield, 141–155.

Deglin, V. (1970), "O lateralizacii mexanizma èmocional'noj okraski povedenija," *Farmakologičeskie osnovy antidepressionogo povedenija,* Leningrad, 158–162.

Deglin, V., & N. Nikolaenko (1975), "O roli dominantnogo polušarija v reguljacii èmocional'nyx sostojanij čeloveka," *Fiziologija čeloveka* 1, 418–426.

Eggert, G. H. (1977), *Wernicke's Works on Aphasia: A Sourcebook and Review,* The Hague.

Gainotti, Guido (1972), "Emotional behavior and hemispheric side of the lesion," *Cortex* 8, 41–55.

Galaburda, A. M., M. LeMay, T. L. Kemper, & Norman Geschwind (1978), "Right-Left Asymmetries in the Brain," *Science* 199, 852–856.

Gates, Anne, & J. L. Bradshaw (1977), "Music Perception and Cerebral Asymmetries," *Cortex* 13, 390–401.

Gazzaniga, M. S. (1970), *The bisected brain*, New York.

Gazzaniga, M. S., & R. W. Sperry (1967), "Language after Section of the Cerebral Commissures," *Brain* 90, 131–148.

Geschwind, N. (1967), "Wernicke's Contribution to the Study of Aphasia," *Cortex* 3, 449–463.

——— (1979), "Specializations of the Human Brain," *Scientific American* 3, 180–199.

Halliday, A. M., K. Davidson, M. W. Browne, & L. C. Kreeger (1968), "Comparisons of the Effects on Depression and Memory of Lateral E.C.T. and Unilateral E.C.T. to the Dominant and Non-Dominant Hemispheres," *British Journal of Psychiatry* 114, 997–1012.

Ivanov, Vjačeslav V. (1978), *Čet i nečet; asimmetrija mozga i znakovyx sistem*, Moscow.

——— (1979), "Nejrosemiotika ustnoj reči i funkcional'naja asimmetrija mozga," *Acta et Commentationes Universitatis Tartuensis* 481, 121–142.

Jackson, J. H. (1958), *Selected Writings*, ed. by J. Taylor, II, New York.

Jakobson, R. (1962), *Selected Writings* I, The Hague.

——— (1971), *Selected Writings* II, The Hague.

——— (1980), *The Framework of Language*, Ann Arbor.

Jakobson, R., & L. Waugh (1979), *The Sound Shape of Language*, Bloomington, Ind. and London.

Kimura, D. (1961), "Cerebral Dominance and the Perception of Verbal Stimuli," *Canadian Journal of Psychology* 15, 166–171.

Kimura, D. (1964), "Left-Right Differences in the Perception of Melodies," *Quarterly Journal of Experimental Psychology* 16, 355–358.

King, F. L., & D. Kimura (1972), "Left-Ear Superiority in Dichotic Perceptions of Vocal Nonverbal Sounds," *Canadian Journal for Psychology* 26, 111–116.

Knox, C., & D. Kimura (1970), "Cerebral Processing of Nonverbal Sounds in Boys and Girls," *Neuropsychologia* 8, 227–237.

Luria, A. R. (1973), "Two Basic Kinds of Aphasic Disorders," *Linguistics* 115, 57–66.

______ (1974), "Language and Brain: Towards the Basic Problems of Neurolinguistics," *Brain and Language* 1, 1–14.

______ (1977), "The Contribution of Linguistics to the Theory of Aphasia," *Roman Jakobson—Echoes of His Scholarship,* ed. by D. Armstrong & C. H. van Schooneveld, Lisse, 237–251.

Maruszewski, M. (1975), *Language Communication and the Brain,* The Hague.

Milner, B. (1962), "Laterality Effects in Audition," *Interhemispheric Relations and Cerebral Dominance,* ed. by V. B. Mountcastle, Baltimore, 177–195.

______ (1975), "Hemispheric Specialization: Scope and Limits," *Hemispheric Specialization and Interaction,* ed. by B. Milner, Cambridge, Mass., 75–88.

Mindadze, A. A., V. M. Mosidze, & T. D. Kakuberi (1975), "O muzykal'noj funkcii pravogo polušarija mozga čeloveka," *Communications of the Georgian Academy of Sciences* 79, 457–459.

Monrad-Krohn, G. M. (1947), "Dysprosody or Altered Prosody in Language," *Brain* 70, 405–415.

Osolsobě, I. (1967), "Ostension as the Limit Form of Communication and Its Significance in Art," *Estetika* 14, Prague, Czech paper 2–23 with an English summary.

Peirce, Charles Sanders (1958), *Collected Papers* II and IV, ed. by A. W. Burks, Cambridge, Mass.

Peuser, G. (1977), *Sprache und Gehirn: Eine Bibliographie zur Neurolinguistik*, Munich.

Sapir, Edward (1949), *Selected Writings*, Berkeley and Los Angeles.

Sperry, R. W. (1975), "Lateral Specialization in the Surgically Separated Hemispheres," *Hemispheric Specialization and Interaction*, ed. by B. Milner, Cambridge, Mass., 5–19.

Trubetzkoy, N. S. (1939), *Grundzüge der Phonologie = Travaux du Cercle Linguistique de Prague* 7; English translation by C.A.M. Bultaxe (1969), *Principles of Phonology*, U. of California Press.

Wolf, Catherine G., & Elissa Koff (1978), "Memory for Pure and Verb-Derived Nouns: Implications for Hemispheric Specialization," *Brain and Language* 5, 36–41.

RECENT BOOKS BY R. JAKOBSON

Six leçons sur le son et le sens, Paris, Editions de Minuit, 1976—*Six Lectures on Sound and Meaning*, Hassocks (Eng.), Harvester Press, and Cambridge, Mass., MIT Press, 1978—*Sei lezioni sul suono e sul senso*, Milano, Il Saggiatore, 1978—*Seis lições sobre o som e o sentido*, Lisbon, Moraes Editores, 1977—*Oto to Imi ni tsuite no Rokusho*, Tokyo, Misuzu Shobo, 1977.

[with Linda Waugh] *The Sound Shape of Language*, Bloomington, Indiana University Press, and Hassocks (Eng.), Harvester Press, 1979—*La Charpente phonique du langage*, Paris, Editions de Minuit, 1980.

The Framework of Language, prefaced by L. Matejka, Ann Arbor, Michigan Studies in the Humanities, 1980.

Elementer, funktioner og strukturer i sproget, Copenhagen, Nyt Nordisk, 1979.

N. S. Trubetzkoy's Letters and Notes, annotated edition, The Hague, Mouton, 1975.

[with Krystyna Pomorska] *Dialogues*, Paris, Flammarion, 1980.

Selected Writings V: On Verse, Its Masters and Explorers, ed. by Stephen Rudy, The Hague, Mouton, 1979—*Selected Writings III: Poetry of Grammar and Grammar of Poetry*, ed. by Stephen Rudy, The Hague, Mouton, to appear.

Questions de poétique, revised edition, Paris, Editions du Seuil, 1978—*Ensayos de Poética*, Mexico, Fondo de Cultura Economica, 1977—*Poetik: Ausgewählte Aufsätze 1921–1971*, ed. by Elmar Holenstein, Frankfurt, Suhrkamp, 1978—*Ogledi iz Poetike*, introduced by Leon Kojen, Beograd, Prosveta, 1978.

[with Stephen Rudy] *Yeats' "Sorrow of Love" Through the Years*, Lisse, Peter de Ridder Press, 1977.

Hölderlin—Klee—Brecht: Zur Wortkunst dreier Gedichte, Frankfurt, Suhrkamp, 1976—*Hölderlin, l'arte della parola*, Genova, Il Melangolo, 1979.

Langage enfantin et aphasie, Paris, Flammarion, 1980.

Lo sviluppo della semiotica, Milano, Bompiani, 1978.